Preface;

My name is Delinda Rodgers, the mother of the little girl, Lacey Rodgers, who will be the subject of this story. I'm writing this book, because I feel like the Lord wants me to tell about the marvelous things He was willing to do for our family, during the time that our daughter Lacey, was sick with leukemia, took her chemo, and recovered from the cancer that came into her life, like it does to so many other wonderful children. I feel like God would want me to share this with other families that are, and might be going through what we went through during this very difficult time.

I know in my heart, God lead us to this cross for a purpose, and that purpose was to get my husband Greg, and myself, closer to Him, and to teach us to depend on Him, for all things. When God leads us to our cross, and when He leads you to your cross, no matter how big or how small that cross may be, I can assure you, it will be;

"The Perfect Cross".

I do hope you enjoy reading this book as much as I enjoyed writing it.

The Author: Delinda Rodgers

INDEX:

Chapter 1.
What is wrong with our Lacey?

Sometime during the month of September 2C my mother, Thelma Stevens, became a little concern about the color of Lacey's skin. (Lacey is my daught and this story is about her, and something awful and wonderful, that happened to her). She, my moth thought she had a little bit of a yellow tint to her. I did think anything about it and passed it off as her losing 1 summer tan.

The week of Halloween, a friend of ours cal and asked if Lacey could play catchers position for t team that was playing in Tulsa, in a Hallowe tournament. They were one player short of having a f team, they promised all of the tournament fees would covered, and Lacey really wanted to play. They play several games, 2 or 3, and I remember between gam she just laid on our laps, she seemed so worn out a tired, no energy, just plain run down.

Halloween night we took the girls trick treating, but Lacey didn't act right, she wasn't runni from house to house like she normally would have bee After about 20 or 30 minutes she was done and ready go home, which didn't make Sarah, that is Lace sister, very happy.

The Thursday before Thanksgiving Lacey came home from school very tired, run down and running just a slight fever, nothing real alarming. I told her she was probably coming down with a bug of some sort, and that she probably would be ok by the time school started back up after thanksgiving break. So, she got one extra day for break than the rest of the kids. Well, she wasn't any better, and she wasn't any worse, just not any better, and that worried me. We had gone on to church as we figured whatever she had was not contagious because Greg and Sarah had not caught it yet, and they catch everything.

This was before we took her to the hospital.

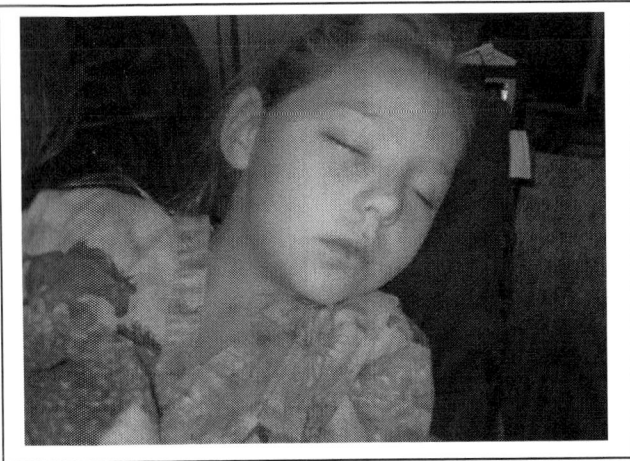

Her skin was becoming more and more yellow it seemed like it anyway, more so each and every day. After church one Sunday Sis. Barbara Morris, told me that I might do some research on Mono. One of her children had mono when they were younger and that they had a lot of the same symptoms that Lacey had so, when we got home I got on the internet and looked up mono and it's symptoms. That was it! She had mono. I called the school the next morning and told the principal what I thought she had. He knew about our religious beliefs, about not going to the doctors and gave us no problems about it. He told me that they wouldn't expect her back then till after Christmas break. He said he knew that even with treatment that mono is a type of disease that has to run it's course, and that takes 6 to 8 weeks.

From Thanksgiving break to December 10, 2005 things seemed to be the same. She had no appetite, tired all the time, no energy and a slight fever 99.8 to 100.2 nothing real alarming. Lacey was staying with my Mom and Dad a lot. Because Greg was working, Sarah and I were going to school. I was taking a business computer course at Central Tech in Drumright.

On Sunday December 11th, Lacey wanted to spend the night with Papa and Nana. During the night my Dad, Durward Stevens, woke and noticed there was a light on in the bathroom and heard a noise coming from inside. Dad knocked on the door, and said Lacey's name. Lacey said, "come in Papa,"

He went in and found her fully dressed setting on the lid of the toilet crying. Dad asked her why she was crying and why she didn't wake him. She said, "Oh Papa, you were sleeping and I didn't want to disturb you." Dad invited Lacey to sleep with him and Nana. Lacey loves to cuddle while sleeping. So Dad didn't have to twist her arm too much.

By the next morning Dad and Lacey's pajamas were soaked from Lacey running just enough of a fever to cook Dad through the night. Mom and Dad got up and left Lacey to sleep for a while. About 11am Mom and Dad decided it was time she woke up. They both went in and kissed her till she woke up. Then Mom fixed her a bowl of cereal. While she was trying to eat, she was having problems holding on to the spoon. She asked, "Nana, why can't I hold on to my spoon, I keep dropping it on the table"? Nana told her she probably slept on it wrong and that her hand and arm was probably asleep. We could hardly get her to eat much; little bites here and there were about it. After a few bites of her cereal she decided she was done. She was quickly dwindling away to nothing, and her little legs looked like toothpicks. Anyway Mom sent her to the bathroom to brush her teeth. While brushing her teeth she was still having problems holding on to anything. She just couldn't keep the toothbrush in her hand. Mom went to the bathroom to check on Lacey, then went to the living room and told Dad, "Durward, there is something

seriously wrong with this baby!" Just as Dad stepped into the bathroom Lacey collapsed. Dad caught her and kept her from hitting the floor, and said, "Oh Lord have mercy." He carried her to the couch and then called for the elders of the church, at Sapulpa. Mom called me, and I was on my lunch break catching up on laundry and dishes. I answered the phone, as Mom says, "Delinda, don't panic, but we think Lacey has just had a stroke."
I hung up the phone and called Greg crying. He was working in Cushing and as I tell him what's going on, he drops his tool belt, and tells the guy he's working with, "I've gotta go." And he heads to Mom and Dads.

On my way to my Mom and Dads, which is 6.5 miles East of Drumright on Highway 33. I'm praying, begging God to spare my baby girl. I was the first to arrive, and by the time I got there, the Lord has already answered my prayers. I walked in, and she's setting up on the couch and smiling BIG at me, and saying, "Mommy!" as I go to her, I drop to my knees and cry out in prayer, thanking God for his mercy. Mom and Dad are crying, I'm crying, and Lacey is happy! She was 8 years old at the time and not understanding just how serious all of this was. Greg gets there, walks through the door, and I'm still on my knees hugging Lacey, crying and praying. He kneels down beside me and I let him hold her for a while. He's crying and thanking God too, for having mercy on her. Shortly after Greg got there, Bro. James Morris and Bro. Dewayne Hale came in. Greg and I made way for the elders to get to her, as they kneel down in front of her and began to pray for her one at a time.

After they prayed, they anointed her with olive oil, and prayed for her again. Mom and Dad began to tell all of us, what Lacey had done and how she had acted. The right side of her face was drawn up, and back, and she couldn't use the right side of her body very well. She couldn't concentrate long enough to put a full sentence together or even say her ABC's. We all decided that it surely did sound like a stroke.

After the elders left, I got on the Internet to look up the symptoms of mono again. I told Greg, "I don't know what this is, but it's not mono! Nowhere does it talk about having strokes with mono."

We were home before 3 pm, so we would be there when Sarah got off the bus from school. We called several people to tell them what had happened to Lacey earlier that day, so they would know to be praying for her.

For the next few days everything seemed to go ok she didn't seem to be affected by the stroke, but then 4 days after the 1st stroke came the 2nd stroke. It was on the 16th of December, I can't remember why, but she was with me at my school, and everyone knew she'd been sick and my teacher didn't mind her being there with me. She didn't feel good so she lay under my desk and slept most of the day. I'm sure there were a few of my classmates that didn't even know she was there. When it was time for class to be over I handed in my assignment, woke Lacey up and got ready to go. I was folding her blanket and she says, "Mommy, It's happening again." I said, "Ok baby, let's hurry up and get out of here before someone notices that there is something wrong." I had to practically carry her to the truck because her right leg wouldn't work. When we got home, I had her to stay in the truck, and I went to call Greg and Mom & Dad, and they called the elders for me. I was to meet Greg and the elders out at Mom and Dads. By the time I got Lacey out there, she had come out of it and seemed to be doing ok. Greg got there and prayed for her, then Bro. James Morris and Bro. Bill Grady got there and they prayed for her. God had mercy and she didn't seem to be effected by the 2nd stoke. All her limbs worked ok, and she could count and say her ABC's fine. Four days later she had a 3rd stroke. This time she was with Greg. He was home from work so she stayed with him while I went to school. I can't remember what time it was but Greg called my school and said. "Get home NOW! She's doing it again." I'm sure I had a funny look on my face because Mrs. Frank never said a word to me when I went flying out of the room with not even an explanation. I hollered over my shoulder for someone to put my things away for me and I was out of there. When I walked through the door Greg was setting on the couch, beside her, praying and crying. He looked up at me and said, "She just now come out of it." She said, "Mommy, this was the worst one yet." Once again I knelt before my baby and begged God to have mercy. Mom and Dad came and prayed and then Bro. James and Bro. Bill Grady came and prayed and God had mercy. Once again she seemed to be unaffected by the stroke.

Later that night before we went to bed Greg and I were talking about how we felt about what was going on with Lacey. We decided we needed to pray together, so we knelt down beside our bed and poured our hearts out to God. We had been doing this almost every night since Lacey first started getting sick, and I remember Greg's prayer that night because he prayed that God would make an opportunity to visit Carlos on the job. Greg worked for Bro. Carlos Combs doing construction work.

The next day was the 20th of December, (my last day of school) While working, out of the blue, Carlos brought up the subject of Lacey being sick. He asked Greg if he was prepared to deal with the consequences if Lacey should die. Carlos told Greg that both he and I would probably be put in jail and Sarah would be put into foster care. That hit Greg hard! He couldn't handle the thought of Lacey dying, not to mention Sarah being put in foster care and me being put in jail. When Greg got home that night he told me what he and Carlos had talked about. We both got down and prayed for answers of what God wanted us to do. Greg had called a couple of different ministers, to ask them exactly where in the Bible it reads, that it's wrong to go to the doctor. The ministers gave him the scriptures he was seeking for, he read and read and reread. We went into a fast seeking God for a sign, or for Him to lead someone to talk to us, or something. The next day Greg went to work, Sarah went to school, and I stayed home with Lacey. That evening when Greg got home from work, he said he had something he wanted to talk to me about, so we went to the bedroom and he asked me, "What do you think about taking her to the hospital?" My mouth dropped to the floor. Usually I would've been the first one to mention going to the hospital. Until that Moment I had not realized the amount of peace that God had granted me. Even after this point I continued to feel no panic.

After talking about it for a while we decided to take it to the Lord, and let Him tell us what to do. So, once again we knelt down beside our bed and prayed for an answer, or some sort of sign, so we could know what God wanted us to do.

After we prayed, we walked to the living room, I set on the edge of the couch, and we asked Lacey what she thought about us taking her to the hospital? She began to panic, as she had never been to a hospital and she became frightened. Her eyes welled up with tears and said, "No Momma, I'm scared." I too, started to cry, and said, "I'm scared too baby, but if they can tell us what is wrong with you, maybe we can fix it here at home. It could be something very simple, something that we can feed you, or something that we shouldn't be feeding you."

Just about that time, there was a knock at the door Greg and I dropped our jaw, I answered the door, and there stood my Grandma and Grandpa Overacker. I looked at Greg and said, "Well, here's our answer." But that answer wasn't at all what I thought it would be. You see my grandparents are very strict when it comes to going to the hospital. So, It came as quit a shock, when they told us that they would stand behind us if we chose

11.

to take Lacey to the hospital. Grandma's exact words to me were, "After just loosing Sandra in March, I don't think I could handle loosing another one, so soon."

Chapter 2.
The decision is made

Greg and I were still very unsure what to do. Grandma talked me into letting Sarah go home with them, so if we did decide to take Lacey to the hospital, we wouldn't have to worry about her.

After they left with Sarah, we called Mom and Dad to tell them that grandma and grandpa had just left, and what they had to say. We asked what they're advice to us would be and they had none except to pray about it. Which, we had been, for days. Finally, we decided, we would take her. I had bought the girls a really cute pajama set for Christmas and I asked Lacey, if she would like to open one of her presents tonight. She was all for that. I just thought it would be nice if she had something nice to wear just in case they wanted to admit her into the hospital.

Still unsure if we were doing the right thing, we loaded up into Greg's truck and drove very slowly, still praying that if we were doing the wrong thing, God would make one of the tires go flat, or something before we got to the hospital. It didn't happen, and we drove right to the emergency room, and set in the parking lot for a little while still praying that God would stop us from doing anything he wouldn't be pleased with. It was kind of cool that night but not cold, cold. Lacey had a light throw blanket wrapped around her shoulders. We all walked into the Drumright hospital with Lacey in the middle of Greg and I. As soon as the doctors and nurses saw her they knew by the color of her skin something wasn't right. One of them had mentioned right away "Some sort of Hepatitis" Well I thought, mono is a type of hepatitis.

They could tell she was dehydrated so they started an IV in her left arm and started her on fluids. They also took blood and sent it to the lab for all types of testing. While we waited for testing we called several people for prayers. Mom and Dad had called Aunt Mona and Uncle Buddy and a lot of others to start a prayer line. Also, while we were waiting, which by the way, seemed like hours, James and Paula (Greg's brother and his wife) and Jarrett and Kristy (our oldest son and his wife) came to the Drumright hospital to be with us.

Finally, Dr. Erin Trippy came to the room where we were waiting and asked us to come to a different room to talk. Kristy stayed in the room with Lacey so she wouldn't have to be by herself. I guess the Dr. could tell that we were not Dr. oriented, so she asked Paula to go with us so she could translate information in case we didn't understand what was being said. We weren't use to the language that doctors spoke, as we had been taught all our lives that it was a lack of faith to go to the doctors, so we never went.

Dr. Trippy, Greg, and I and James and Paula and Jarrett went to this little room they called the chapel, we set down and the doctor began to explain to us what she thought was wrong with Lacey. She said it could be one of two things, leukemia or T-cell or something like that

14.

I'm not sure exactly what she said. Paula Instantly started crying. The Doctor said that the Drumright hospital was not properly equipped to treat her and that Saint Francis had the best children's hospital in this area. Greg asked if we could take her in his truck and she said, "Absolutely not!" She began to tell us about her hemoglobin. At Lacey's age her Hemoglobin should be between 12 – 14, the doctors give blood transfusions to people when they're Hemoglobin gets down to 8, hers was 2.5. They said she should not have even been coherent. She should have been in a coma.

On the way to St. Francis hospital, they would only let one person ride in the ambulance. Greg told me to ride with her and he would take the truck behind us, seeing as how, I couldn't see in the dark very well to drive. Jarrett rode with Greg, Kristi took their vehicle, and James and Paula took theirs.

By the time we got to St. Francis it was after midnight. Mom and Dad, my sister and her husband, Robert and Christle and their two boys, Brandon and Matthew, were there, waiting on us.

We went through the ER and then up to the room they had waiting for us. When we got to the room, there were lots of doctors and nurses waiting to ask questions, and hook her up to all kinds of machines. After a while, we did get a break and I went to ask if our family could go back to see her because none of them had seen her yet? They said, "Sure bring them back."

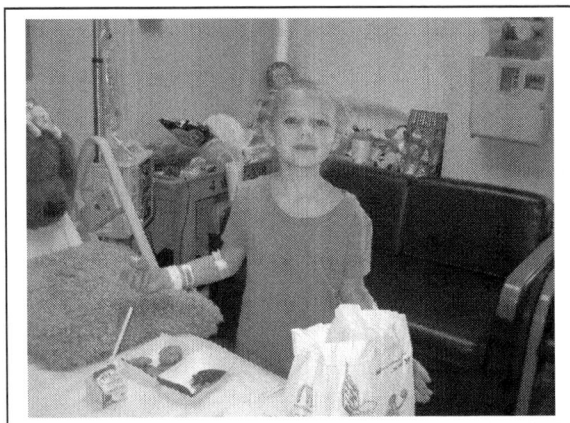

And I said, "ALL of them?" "Yes that will be fine." So, I went to the waiting room to bring them all back. The nurses were standing in the hallway whispering to each other, "That's too many, that's too many." I probably won't be able to name them all, but here we go; two of my Dads sisters, aunt Sonja and aunt Tawana; our oldest son Jarrett and his wife Kristy and little boy, Raider; Our oldest daughter Keidra, and her husband Jeremy; Greg's brother James and his wife Paula. It sure seemed like there were a lot more people there but I can't remember any others.

It was almost 4 o'clock in the morning when we finally laid down to get some sleep. James and Paula stayed all night. James went to his truck to sleep, Greg took the couch, and Paula and I shared the cot they brought for us.

About 3 hours later (7:00 am) the doctor, whom we've grown to love, Dr. Gregory Kirkpatrick, slowly cracked open the door, peeked his head in, with a mask over his mouth and nose. Lacey sets straight up in bed and says, "Excuse me, (which wakes up everyone in the room) are you sure you have the right room?" He replies by saying "well are you Lacey Rodgers?" she says, "yes I am." "Well then, I have the right room, but I like that attitude! Anytime anyone comes in this room, and your not sure if they should be in here, you have every right to question them. Who are you, and what do you want?"

He went on to explain why he had the mask on, he had a slight cold and as low as Lacey's counts were he didn't want to take the chance of giving anything to her. He was a very nice man, and he explained to Lacey, everything that was going on and what they planned on doing to her. I'm sure someone told him of our religion, because he talked to us in very simple terms.

During the next 12 to 24 hours dozens of nurses, doctors, techs and people from the labs came to Lacey's room to see for themselves, that she was in as good of a condition as all the reports had said she was. No one could believe that she was up and moving around her room and playing and laughing, and knew who all of her family members were. She didn't even act like there was anything wrong with her. They told us that her body contains 12 pints of blood, and they gave her 9 pints of blood in 3 days. Everyone thought she should have been in a coma. But she was feeling FABULOUS! Isn't God great?

This was two or three days after we got to the hospital.

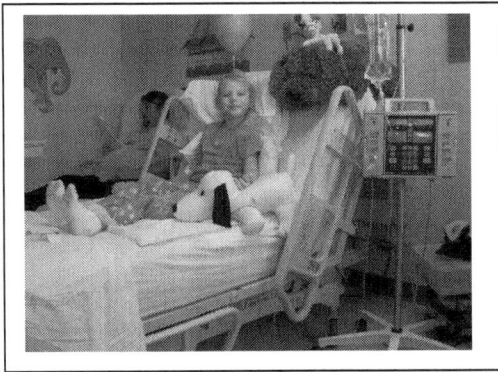

Chapter 3.
A new experience, DOCTORS

We had an enormous amount of visitors! Friends, family, Lots, of church members. People bringing food, drinks, gifts, money, we were so over whelmed with the generosity of everyone. On the 23rd of December 2005, they finally confirmed that she had leukemia. They told us that the type of leukemia she had, was the least aggressive and the easiest to treat. Plus there was an 87% cure rate. The odds were in her favor. They called it, Acute Lymphoblastic Leukemia, it sounds scary, huh? It was. But they set us down, and explained to us just exactly what was involved, and they made it sound, not so scary. God was good to us, and by His grace, we were able to get through it.

They gave us a videotape to watch because they had to have permission to insert a portacath, or port, as they called it. A port, is a little metal bowl that has a plastic tube coming off the bottom of the bowl. The bowl would set under the skin, under her left collarbone. The plastic tube is inserted into one of the main veins going into the heart. The port, is where they would draw all her blood from, and give her chemo. They said, if we chose not to have the port, that would be okay, but all the harsh chemicals they would be giving her for the next 2½ years, would most likely collapse the blood vessels in her arm, then they would have to go into different parts of the body to replace those collapsed blood vessels. The port would be less painful for her in the long run.

We showed the tape to a lot of family members and church friends so that they could understand what the port was used for, and how it would benefit her.

Our oldest daughter and her husband brought Lacey a beautiful little white, fiber-optics Christmas tree, pre lit and pre decorated, to sit on the ledge of her windowsill, plus they also brought other Christmas decorations too. Someone else, I don't remember who it was, brought her a little tree, and we set it in the other widow sill. Her room looked very festive.

CHRISTMAS EVE: Dr. K seriously considered letting us go home for Christmas, then return the day after Christmas. But he was afraid, as bad as her condition was, only 3 days ago, to let her out of sight, so to speak, was scary, so we stayed. You could tell it was the Christmas holiday; people were in the giving mood. Christmas Eve and Christmas Day we had people bringing toys, blankets, decorative pillows, build-a-bears, books, coloring books, crayons, paper, pencils, and all kinds of presents. Not just for Lacey either, they brought stuff for Sarah and even Greg and I. A lot of these people we didn't even know. They had done a toy drive in their community or something like that, and brought those things to the hospital for the children who had to be in the hospital, during the Christmas holidays. A lot of these things also came from our own church members. I remember this cheerleading squad gave out build-a-bears. There were a couple of fire stations that brought things too, and there was this one lady that said, she had a childhood cancer and was in the hospital one Christmas herself and ever since, she had brought things to give away to the children during the Christmas season. We were over whelmed by the generosity and unaware of the need for this type of thing, so it really opened up our eyes.

Christmas evening we had a room full of family members. We were all supposed to go to grandma Overacker's for Christmas dinner and gifts. Everyone but us, got to go, but they made it up to us. They brought us leftovers, and no one opened their gifts, they brought all the gifts to the hospital and opened them with us. It was so special!

Look at that smile, she is one happy little girl.

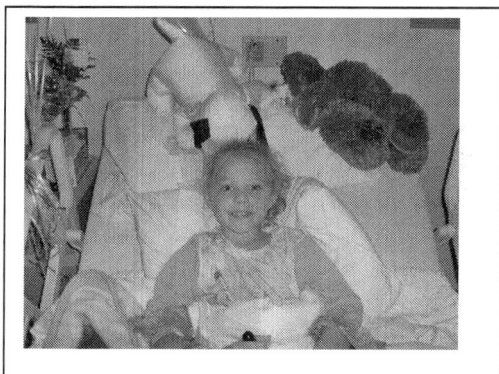

Chapter 4.
Lacey, the unusual girl, to say the least

The nurses said they could tell that Lacey was one loved little girl. She received more visitors than any of their other patients. In fact there were a couple of nurses that told us that sometimes when a child has been admitted to the hospital that the parents don't even come to see them and when the child is released they will call the parents to let them know that they're child is ready to go home. They say this happens to all ages from infants to teens. So they were pretty flabbergasted to see so many people coming to see Lacey.

By the time the evening was over I told Greg teasing, "We're going to have to rent a Uhaul Truck, to get all of these things home."

The day after Christmas Lacey had her first surgery ever. They inserted the port, gave her a spinal tap, which is a really long needle they insert into the core of her spin and extract spinal fluid. (Did you know the spinal fluid is the only fluid in our bodies that is clear? Just a little trivia). Anyway, they also took bone marrow from her hip. The big hip bone in your back, they chip a little hole in the bone and extract marrow from the middle of the bone. OUCH!!!!

She pulled through the surgery like a trooper. In fact she kind of surprised Dr. K that she felt as good as she did. Not an hour after they brought her back to her room, she was up tormenting the nurses with her new remote control truck, she had received for Christmas, from Uncle Robby and Aunt Christle, she was chasing them up and down the hallway.

We asked the doctor, "Should she be up running around so soon after surgery?" He said, "Don't ever stop her from doing what she feels like doing!" He said he himself was blown away at how active she was after just having surgery and her first chemo treatment. Once again, God is good.

The news of Lacey having cancer spread all over the country. We were getting phone calls from everywhere. Mom and Dad were also getting lots of phone calls. Even my sister Christle from Sapulpa and my grandmother from Cushing, was receiving calls. Everyone was so concerned.

One afternoon I got a surprise call from my best friend Heather Combs, who, at the time lived in Colorado. She had heard from her grandmother, but was sure that she had heard wrong, because it was Sarah that had always been our sick child.

When we got home on the 30th of December, our whole town of Drumright knew what was going on. Well, except for the cop that stopped me for speeding. I didn't get a ticket, I told her why I was speeding and she let me off with a warning.

This is what I told the officer, "We just got home from the hospital with our daughter, we found out two days before Christmas that she had leukemia. When we got home today I had forgotten that we had rented movies. Well those movies were late and I was trying to get down to the movie store before they closed to explain why they were late." The officer apologized for our misfortune and sent me on my way.

When I got to the movie store they were just about to close but I caught her at the door locking up, she told me to put the movies in the drop box, I explained to her that it was very important that I talk to her. I told her the whole story and offered to pay the late fees, but the lady told me not to worry about the late fees that she herself would take care of them.

Everyone was so generous to help in any manner they could whether it be taking care of late fees, setting with Lacey to give me an hour or two to myself. Someone even paid our January bills; phone, utilities, and the electric. To this day I still do not know who did that, nor would the utility company tell me who paid them. They told me it was anonymous and they couldn't tell me who it was. The only thing I could do was pray that God would bless whoever done it in a special manner.

Several months before Lacey had gotten sick, something had gone wrong with the car I was driving, so I had to start driving this old clunker that Greg had setting in the yard. It wasn't very dependable but it did get me to school and back home MOST of the time. There were a few times that it did leave me stranded. Anyway, Our oldest daughter, Keidra had a car just like mine, she had rolled her car and the body wasn't in as good a shape as mine so we gave her the car and her husband and his father switched out parts. She felt like she had a new car.

After a while, a few months, Jeremy got her a different car, and that car was just setting in their driveway. When they realized I didn't have a dependable vehicle to take Lacey to her doctors' appointments they gave me the car back. We were so thankful; we had talked about how we were going to manage this. Greg had to work and I had to take her to Tulsa, anywhere from one to four times a week. That car lasted me from January of '06 till February of '08.

I can't remember if school started back on the 2nd or the 3rd but anyway, I took the girls to the school, Sarah was staying, but Lacey could only visit her friends and classmates and teachers. She hadn't been in school for about a month and a half, so she was missing everyone. When we walked through the door it was obvious that everyone knew what was going on. They flocked her like ants on a lollipop. It was great!

Mrs. Paul came to talk to me. Her son Cody had cancer several years ago, and she wanted me to know she knew how I felt and if I ever needed anyone to talk to, she was always there for me. I took Lacey to her classroom so she could see her teacher, Mrs. Erwin, and all her classmates. Lacey told everyone all about her cancer and what the doctors had done to her while she was in the hospital and what she was going to have to do for the next 2½ years. She told them she probably wouldn't be in class for the rest of the year but she would try to come visit if she had a good day. I went to talk to Mr. Hiett, the principal, about me coming to the school and getting a weeks worth of work for her. He told me that would not be necessary that the state of Oklahoma had a home bound program so she wouldn't miss any of her studies, and the program provided a tutor if Lacey needed one, which he didn't suspect that she would, but it was there if she needed it. But, instead of a tutor, Mrs. Erwin thought Lacey would be more comfortable, if she came by the house twice a week to give Lacey her work, and show her how to do what she needed to do. So, for the rest of the school year, Mrs. Erwin was at our house. She would keep Lacey in the loop of what was going on in school, and Lacey really enjoyed seeing Mrs. Erwin when she came.

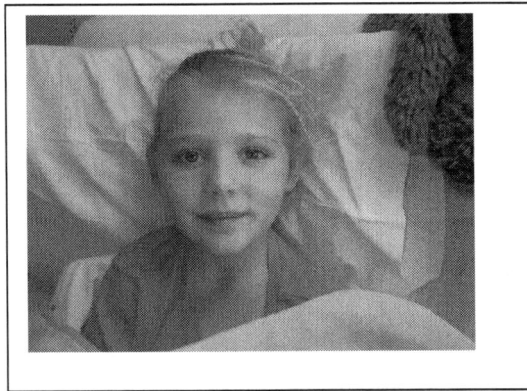

Chapter 5.
The real meaning of FRIENDS

A few days after we were home, Lacey's softball coach, Wyatt Earp, called and wanted to know if we'd be offended if he organized a fund raiser for Lacey, so when she had other hospital visits and Greg was out of work we would be able to make ends meet, or if she needed anything special, or medical expenses that insurance didn't cover, or whatever we wanted to use the money for. We told him he didn't have to do that, but we would not be offended. He insisted that was what he wanted to do. He advertised for weeks, he even got the central tech involved. The printing class made hundreds of flyers announcing "The Chili Supper."

Everyone at the vo-tech knew me, I had been going to school out there for about 2½ - 3 years before Lacey got sick. I had worked the switchboard for close to a month, I helped a few of the teachers with computer programs, so they're students could test online. I had helped some in the main office as well. So I was pretty well known out there and everyone heard about what was going on and that Wyatt was taking up a collection for Lacey they were more than generous. Wyatt had even spoken to all the businesses in town and they too contributed to the fundraiser in some way or another. Some of the people he talked to about Lacey literally emptied their pockets on the spot to donate to the cause.

The word that Wyatt was organizing a fundraiser for Lacey spread quickly and others began to call me to see if they could also do things. One day Lacey's basketball couch, Goldie, called to tell Lacey that they were going to refund the money that we paid for her to play, plus they were having her jersey # put on the sleeves of all the other players in her honor. There were only a few games Lacey felt like going to and rooting for her teammates. She didn't get to play, but she watched from the bench. I don't know if they did this every time, but when we were there most any time, they huddled together, they would break by saying "FOR LACEY."

Meanwhile, during all of this time, Lacey continued her treatments. It only took them 3 weeks to get her into remission. Mind you, the day we walked into the Drumright hospital she only weighed 52 lbs., but 28 days later she weighed 78 lbs. This was caused from the steroids she was taking.

She went from the low figure, to the high figure...in 28 days!!

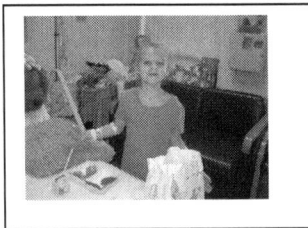

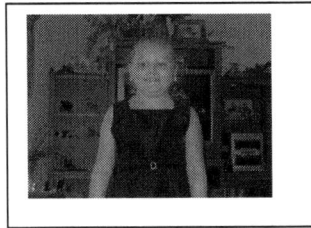

The steroids drove her insane! Bless her heart she just couldn't get full enough. At times she would eat so much she'd look like a little rolly-polly. She'd set and moan for about 30 minutes, still feeling hungry but just simply didn't have any room, then after about 30-45 minutes she'd be in the bathroom getting rid of what she just ate, setting on the toilet, then straight to the refrigerator to make herself miserable again.

I remember one time we were at my Mom and Dads for supper, and after we ate, Lacey asked my mother if she could take the leftovers home so she would have something to eat when we got home, and during the middle of the night. When we got ready to go, we sent the girls out to the car while we were standing at the door, to finish up the last of our conversation and say our good byes. The leftovers didn't make it home. She ate them before we got home, with her hands! Needless to say she needed some cleaning up.

I also remember one time I had told the girls to fold and put away they're clothes, that were on my bed, and as Lacey was changing out of her pajamas, she went to change her under pants and started crying because she couldn't find any that fit. I sat down beside her, put my arm around her and asked her what was wrong, she said, "None of my panties fit me anymore because I've gotten so fat.
I just want to give up!"

Back to the flyers; Wyatt had those flyers made up and gave Bradley school enough to give to every child, one to take home to they're parents. When Walter Hoover saw the flier that Alicia had taken home, he came and hunted Lacey down. He said he had been driving the streets of Drumright trying to find out where she lived. One day we were standing out in the yard and this man, woman, and two kids, pull up and ask my husband, "Do you have any idea where Lacey Rodgers lives?" My husband said, "yes, she lives right here I'm her father." Walter got out of his car and extended his hand out to Greg for a handshake. Greg shook his hand and Walter began to explain to us that he too had leukemia and would like Lacey to know that she's not the only one going through this. We took him into the house, and he set on the edge of the couch, and told Lacey what he'd just told us. He gave her his phone number and told her that if she needed someone to talk to, she could call him anytime.

Walter drove the bus for the Baptist church there in town on Sunday mornings and Wednesday nights. Every time he drove by our house he always honked and waved real big. Him and Lacey became pretty close.

Lacey had been losing her hair pretty bad every time she took a bath the bathtub would be covered in hair and even when she didn't have a bath, and I'd brush her hair so that the hair wouldn't get all over the pillow at night, there was lots of hair that would come out in the brush. I tried to keep as much of it as I could, and I put it in a zip lock bag.

Wyatt scheduled a chili supper for February 2, 2006. When we pulled up into the school parking lot, we were blown away by the amount of people who had shown up. We didn't know half the people that were there. But everyone made us feel so loved. Everyone was so wonderful to us.

Wyatt told us when he would mention to people Lacey's situation and what he was doing to help, people jumped on the band wagon and wanted to be a part of the fundraiser. Danny Davis wanted to make the chili. He told Wyatt that he cooked when he was in the service and knew how to cook for a crowd. There were lots of others that helped, some served the chili, some washed dishes, and after everyone ate, some took money at the door and I don't even know what else. I just know there were a lot of people involved.

The students and faculty of Bradley Elementary had a penny drive for Lacey. They had two jars, one for the boys and one for the girls. They made a contest out of it, and who ever won got some sort of prize. I'm not sure what the prize was, I can't remember. But anyway, the girls ended up winning.

On Valentines Day Lacey had a clinic appointment. They gave her chemo, and then we were on our way. Her hair was so thin, there were places you could clearly see her scalp. I had always told Greg that I didn't want Lacey's hair to look scraggly. On our way home from the clinic we stopped at Mom and Dad's to tell them we had decided to go ahead and cut the rest of her hair off and shave her head to save getting hair all over the place anymore.

Christle and the boys were there and Matthew wanted to shave his head with her, Greg had already told Lacey, that when all her hair was gone he'd shave his head too, so Dad decided he would too. So we had a head shaving party.

After we shaved Lacey's head she really started getting sick. I almost regretted shaving her head. I had even made the comment, "We cut all her Strength off, just like Delilah did to Samson."

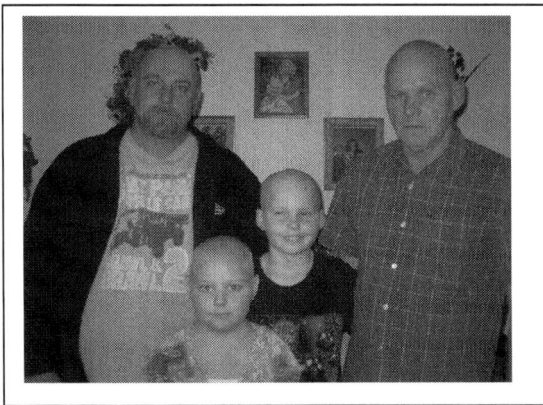

The next day when Matthew went to school, his teacher, from Sapulpa, asked him why he shaved his head in the middle of the wintertime. When he told her that he shaved his head for his cousin, he told her all about Lacey. She was so moved by the jester that she got their school involved in a fundraiser for Lacey.

They had done the pop tabs, and on their last day of school, they had a talent show. They invited us to come, and hoped Lacey would also feel good enough that day, to make it. It turned out that Lacey did feel good that day. We didn't tell them we were coming we wanted it to be a surprise. We walked in a little late. There again we didn't know anyone but because of the flier that Matt had taken to his school to show everyone who Lacey was, everyone already knew her.

When we got there Matthew took Lacey to his teacher to introduce them. Mrs. Speers, and Mrs. Luker, took Lacey to the front of gym, to introduce her to the whole school. Like I said, they were having a talent show and they asked Lacey if she wanted to do something. She just happen to have her Hilary Duff CD, and had been practicing a song. So they put the CD in and she sang, "Someone's Watching Over Me". All the teachers were crying. Christle said that the principal had to walk out of the gym to contain himself, so needless to say, it was successful.

Chapter 6.
Humor, and oh yes, BASEBALL

It was time for softball sign-ups again, and we weren't even sure if Lacey was going to feel like playing that year, but she wanted to signup anyway, just in case. One of the first questions Lacey asked the doctor when she was diagnosed was, "Am I going to get to play softball?" Dr. K said, "You can do anything you feel like doing. But, you're probably not going to feel like playing." She proved him wrong!

They were having softball signups at our local café, called Jo's Drive-In. That year the girls were on the same team. They didn't charge me for Lacey, I think because they didn't think she would be playing much, if any at all.

Jamie Osterhout, was the girls couch that year. Lacey missed every practice from being too sick to raise her head off the pillow.

It was really weird though, Lacey was sick, it seemed like almost every day, but the doctors and nurses rarely ever seen her at her worst. Most of the times when Lacey had clinic appointments, she felt really good. While some of the other children didn't have the energy to walk back to the treatment rooms from the waiting room, Lacey was skipping up and down the hallways and being goofy.

There was this one time, she had to have a blood transfusion and a certain type of chemo that they call the PEGS. It stands for something but I'm not sure what. We don't know if it was a bad reaction to the blood, or the PEGS or a combination of the two, but her lips turned wrong side out, she started throwing up and passing blood through her bowels. She broke out in a rash that ran from her eyebrows, over the top of her baldhead, both ears, down her back to her tailbone. The rash on her back was shaped like a butterfly across her shoulders. It scared me so bad!

I thought we were going to lose her right there. And, I think it kind of shook up the doctors and nurses too, but they tried real hard not to show it because I was already panicked. I called Greg crying, he was working in Cushing, I told him what was going on, so he went from Cushing to St. Francis hospital in Tulsa in 35 minutes. Needless to say he was flying low. I think we were in the hospital for about 4 days that time. Poor little Sarah was shuffled here and there a lot the first 6 months that Lacey was taking chemo.

Lacey kept her humor throughout all of this, as I remember one day we were heading home from one of her clinic visits, it was cool enough outside that I didn't have to run the air conditioner in the car so we had our windows rolled down. We were driving along listening to the radio when all of a sudden Lacey says to me with her head sticking out of the window, "Look Mom, the wind is blowing through my hair!" She was slick bald. I almost had to pull the car over to the side of the road because I was laughing so hard, and I could hardly see from all the tears flowing down my face.

One day when we were at the clinic, and some organization was there, asking some of the kids to paint on unfired ceramic plates. The plates would be auctioned off at a gala, and the proceeds from the gala would be donated to cancer research. The children were to paint a picture that represented one of the months of the year. Lacey chose May. She painted beautiful flowers on the plate. It was so cute. After they had the plates fired that organization brought the plates back to the hospital to show the children how their plate turned out, and all of the pates were so beautiful! The people who bought the plates, went to the gala to entertain some unexpected company that had come in to visit them. They had already discussed it, and had decided they WERE NOT going to bid on anything. After the couple and their friends were finished eating and waiting for the auction to start, the gentlemen walked around to take a look at what all was for auction. When the husband came back to the table where his wife and her friend were visiting, the husband told his wife that they had just bought a set of twelve plates. She told him, "how could you have just bought them the auction hasn't even stared yet." He said. "I don't care what I have to pay for these plates, I'm not walking out of here without them."

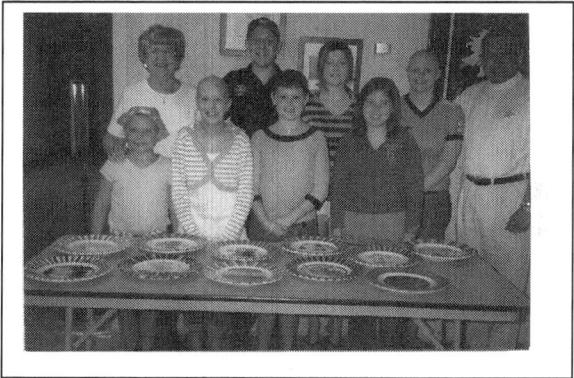

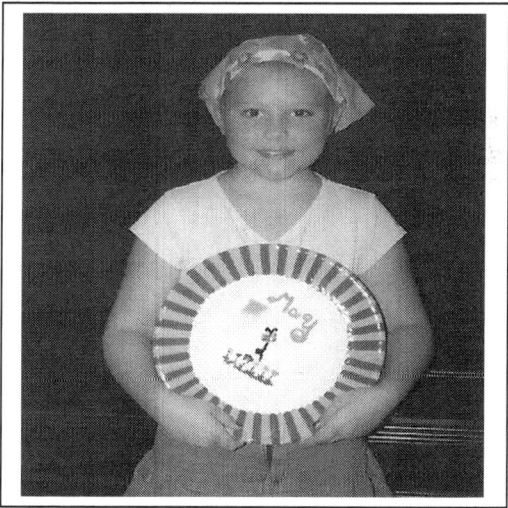

I can't remember what all they said was up for auction but I do remember that there was one of Elvis Presley's signed guitars for auction. Anyway, my point to all of this is, there was a lot of stuff for auction that could have and probably should have went for more than twelve plates! This man took those plates home for the grand price of $9000.00.

A couple of months after the gala was over Lacey asked her nurse Terri, if there would be anyway she could meet the people that bought the plates, so that these people, would be able to put a face with the name on the plate. Terri thought that was a very good idea and was going to talk to all of the parents of the children that painted plates to see if they too would be interested in meeting the people. Jana got in contact with the people to see if they would be interested in meeting the children who painted on the plates, and they loved the idea! So, Jana organized a pizza party there at the hospital. These people surprised the kids and gave the plates back to them. They decided that the kids and the parents would probably enjoy the plates more than they would. So now we have a $750.00 plate hanging on our wall.

Softball is in full swing and so far Lacey hasn't missed one game. I remember this one particular game day; Lacey had a scheduled clinic visit. She had a spinal tap and 4 different types of chemo. After her appointment she was very sore, like she always was after a spinal tap. I called her coach, Jamie Osterhout, to tell him I didn't think she was going to get to play that night. He told me he remembered me telling him at the last game, that she had a spinal tap, so he had already taken her off the batting schedule. Well the longer the day went on the better she got to feeling. She begged me, "Please Momma, I really wanna play, I feel good!" I told her, "sissy, you just had a spinal tap! There's no way you're going to feel like playing two games tonight!" She plays catchers position, so she's up, down, up, down all throughout the whole game. She begs, "Mom please, I feel good. I really wanna play, please?" I said, "Okay here's what we'll do, you suit up, we'll talk to Jamie when we get to Cleveland, if he doesn't think it's a good idea you can set the bench and cheer for your teammates.

When we got to the game, and I ask Jamie what he thought about her playing that night, he says to me, "Are you serious? Do you think that's a good idea?" I told him, "Well she really wants to play, and she says she feels real good. I'm not sure if she should play or not, but you watch your child dwindle away to nothing and this is what gets her up and motivated, I can't tell her no, you tell her no." He looked at me kind of funny and says, "Ok, well, I guess she's going to play." And she did too, all evening long; she played her little heart out.

She made a double play that night, the batter bunted the ball, the pitcher picked it up, tossed it to Lacey and she got the 3rd base runner out, then she threw the ball to the 1st baseman and got the batter out. That was the 3rd out of that inning.

That same night Lacey was on 2nd base, and Sarah come up to bat and Lacey says to Sarah, "Come on sissy, bring me home." For some reason that hit Jim Martin really hard. He's one of the other softball players' Dads and also the President of our local bank. He had to walk away from the crowd to contain himself, and his wife Shelly told us that he was so tender hearted.

After the game was over, Lacey started getting sick. All the way home she'd hold her mouth and tell Greg to pull over because she needed to throw up. She threw up all night long. I asked her, "Sis, was it worth it?" She said, "Yep, every minute of it."

The doctors and nurses, one nurse in particular, couldn't believe we were even letting her play ball. They thought that she might get hurt, mainly at her port area, or over heat or something. I reminded them what they told me about letting her do what she felt like doing, and then they said, "yes, but we were not expecting her to feel like playing." I told them, "When it comes to Lacey you need to expect the unexpected." As I said earlier, the doctors didn't see Lacey as sick as what we did. Every time she went to the clinic and she wasn't as sick as they thought she should be, then they would up her dose of chemo, till finally, they had her maxed out by law.

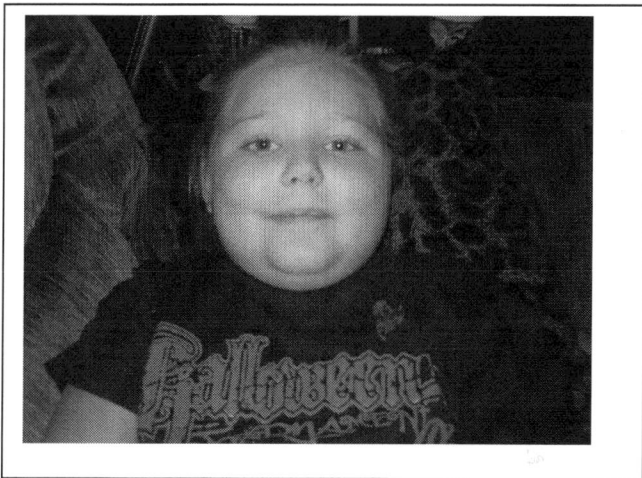

Chapter 7.
You never know, what will happen?

During the 60's they started what they call, THE STUDY. All the blood work they did on Lacey would be documented and compared to other children's blood work. This way they could determine which drug works best for each individual. I'm not sure if it is the types of blood that certain ones have, or just a difference in their chemistry, or what it is. You see, what they didn't seem to understand was that we had a HUGE prayer line going at all times. Every church in Drumright had Lacey on they're prayer list, we didn't go around asking these churches to put her on they're prayer list, but the people that Lacey had come into contact with, would ask us, "Can I put Lacey on our prayer list at my church?" I would say, "Well sure, we can't get too many prayers." Plus we had people from our church, from coast to coast, praying for Lacey also.

One Sunday morning in church at Sapulpa, there was a lady there, from Colorado, Sis. Susan Shamburg, who felt to lay hands on Lacey, then she spoke a command over her, to be made hold. Before this command was spoken, Lacey would wake up 3 or 4 days a week throwing up awful stuff, from her stomach. She might not be sick but just a few hours but then, after that she might have woke up a time or two throwing up, but not very often.

Lacey truly believed in her heart that God healed her that day and she told me she just felt different. She refused to take her medication after that, and for 2 weeks she didn't take it. On the first week I guess there was still enough drugs in her system that it didn't show up in her blood work. But then after the second week, oh boy did we ever get a chewing. They demanded to know why we were not giving her the medication, and that if we chose not to give her the meds, they would get a court order.

We set Lacey down after we got home from the clinic and explained to her what we were going to need to do. Every night before Lacey took her meds, we got down, as a family, in a circle, with Lacey's pills in her hand and took turns praying that God would allow the meds to show up in her blood work, but yet, shield her from the side affects that the pills would normally have. That's exactly what happened, as Lacey very rarely was sick at this point but yet the meds did show up in the blood work.

Chapter 8.
WOW, make a wish, not yet!

I'm not exactly sure what the day or even the month was, but there was a couple that live here in Drumright, Chris and Beth, and they came to our house to make arrangements for Lacey's make-a-wish. Wow, Lacey decided she wanted to go to Disney World, to see Bell, who was on "Beauty and the Beast". We decided we wanted to wait until Lacey was on maintenance to go, so she wouldn't be so sick. So, they scheduled our trip for sometime during the first part of June of 2007.

Sometime during the month of June, a lady from the hospital, Jana Banana, the lady who organized the pizza party, she knew Lacey LOVED softball, and she asked her if she would be interested in throwing out the first pitch at one of the Drillers games? Lacey was so excited. She nearly started to scream! The hospital gave her just so long, to sell tickets to family members and friends, who wanted to see Lacey pitch. The tickets were different prices depending on whether or not you wanted a meal. The hospital said Lacey sold more tickets than anyone had ever sold, 86 tickets to be exact. We had a blast at the Drillers game, as we had never been to a big boys game before. When we first got there, we didn't even get to eat, because they needed Lacey on the field right then!

Greg went down on the field with her and I went up into the stands to shoot video. When they announced her name over the loud speakers, everyone in our group cheered. She walked to the pitchers mound, as I'm video taping, and she throws the ball, I get so excited, I missed the whole thing. But I did get some cool video of the sky. I know, you think I'm an idiot, but anyway we had a blast. The Drillers won the game and at the end of the game, they had a really cool fireworks show.

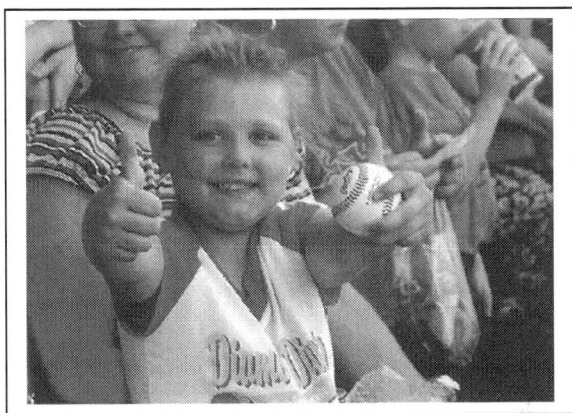

Three days after the Drillers game, the girls start softball camp. The camp was during the day, four hours, and for four days. They allowed me to stay and observe, and there were several other parents that stayed to watch they're kids too. Lacey's hair was really starting to grow out again it was about 2½ to 3" long. On the 1st day about half way through, Lacey pulls off her hat to wipe the sweat from her forehead and when she does, she notices that her hat is full of hair. She asks the instructor if she can come talk to me.

She runs off the field almost in a panic and shows me the inside of her hat. She starts to cry and buries her face in my shoulder; I take her to the bathroom and began to console her. "Sissy, it's okay, they told us that this would probably happen again. It's okay, calm down. Besides that, this way you'll be a lot cooler." "Hay yah you're right, cool!"

She started to calm down, I took a wet cold paper towel and wiped what I could off her head. Most of the rest of the hair that was on her head came off onto the towel.

While I was cleaning her up, the wife of the camp coach, came to check, to make sure Lacey was all right. I let her into the bathroom with us, and then showed her the hat and the paper towel. She gave Lacey a huge hug, and told her that if she wanted to go home for the day and come back the next day, she would tell Brian what was going on. She said, "No thank you, I'd like to finish."

Before we left the bathroom, I wet a towel, and put it on top of Lacey's head. Then I rinsed her hat off and put the hat on top of the towel. We went outside and I told her I wanted to put some more sunscreen on her. I'm pretty sure Brian's wife told him what was going on because I seen him talking to Lacey off away from the other girls. I could see her knotting her head yes, and then no and then yes again. This went on for a few minutes; finally Lacey went on doing what the rest of the girls were doing. She went the rest of the day and never complained a bit. It was the same on the 2nd, 3rd, and 4th day, not one complaint.

At the end of the 4th day the coach handed out T-shirts to all the girls. Then, he handed out just a few trophies. I don't remember who all got trophies or what the trophies were for but they gave one to Lacey for "Best over all." She was on cloud nine!

The doctors told us from the beginning, that the first 6 months of chemo would be the worst, and for the most part it was. But we realize now, that had it not been for God having so much mercy, it could have been so much worse. It probably should have been a lot harder, but she made it easier than it should have been, because she had such a marvelous attitude.

It was getting toward the end of the 6 months and they were going to put her on what they call maintenance for two years. But, before they could put her on maintenance, they had to give her one last big blast of really super hard chemo. For four days they gave her a certain type of chemo, I don't recall the name. They said that after she was done with these four days of chemo, they were going to give her body 2 weeks to recuperate. The chemo they were giving her during these four days was very hard on the body and would drain her of every ounce of energy she had. They also told me that sometime during these two weeks, she would HAVE to have a blood transfusion or platelets or both. (Platelets is what causes your blood to clot) They said, there were a lot of children that had to have both blood, and platelets.

I made up my mind right then and there, that Lacey would not have to have either. I went home, got on my hands and knees, and went into a fast. I begged

God to show his hand in this matter and to prove to those doctors that Lacey was different and that it did not HAVE to be the way they said it would be. I called several family members, and church members to get a prayer line started.

During the two-week break, she did get pretty sickly looking, and pretty drained, and she could hardly eat. But, she slept quite a bit, and she also had zero energy. Her lips got chalky white, but I continued to pray and beg God for this miracle that I was asking for. Everyone I talked to, I would beg them to pray, and I know they did.

On her next clinic appointment we went into the clinic so they could test her blood to see if she needed a transfusion. She was right on the boarder line of needing both. They left the decision up to me and I turned to Lacey knowing that she knew everyone was praying for a miracle." What do you think, Sis?" "Nope, not yet." She said.

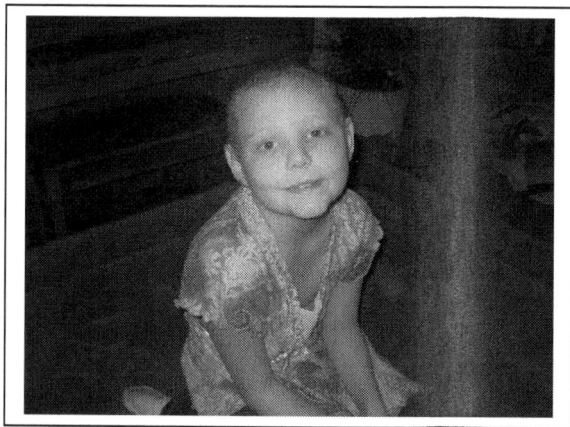

Chapter 9.
See how sickly her eyes look?

One week down one to go. Still everyone continued praying. By the end of the second week Lacey began to recover. She was getting stronger, she was eating better, and her color was coming back to her face.

When we went in for them to check her blood on the 2nd week they just knew that she would probably have to have both blood and platelets because of how poorly she looked last week. When they seen how much she'd improved, they couldn't believe it. When they checked her blood levels, they found out that her body was on it's way to recovery.

One of the nurses said, " Leave it to Lacey to be different, and break all the rules!" They told us, that every child since the 1960's has had to have one or the other or both, but Lacey has made history. The doctor began to ask us all sorts of questions, if we were giving her some sort of vitamins or something. We told them "No, we give her what you tell us to give her and other than that we do A LOT of praying." "Well whatever you're doing keep it up, because it's working."

School was starting and she was so excited! She was still very bald. As a rule the students weren't allowed to wear hats inside the school building. Lacey became spoiled very quickly. She found that it was difficult for most everyone to tell her NO. I discouraged this as much as possible but it didn't do much good. Kids are going to be kids and they will do just exactly what they are allowed to do. I was starting to see something develop in Lacey that I wasn't sure I liked too much. So, I set Lacey down and had a long talk with her about the way she was using her sickness against people, to get what she wanted out of them, and that was not fair. She began to cry, she wasn't even aware that this was what she was doing. After that, I noticed her catching herself doing it, and she would correct herself.

A couple of months after school started Lacey's hair was starting to grow out. A lot of times after she had a shower she would stand in front of the mirror and play with her hair. Trying new styles with her new hair. One time she came out of the bathroom, it was so funny; she had her hair pulled up into a Mohawk. Now mind you, her hair was only 1 to 1½" long. So it didn't stick up to high. The next day she went to school and asked her principal, Mr. Hiett, if she could wear it in a Mohawk to school. He told her that would be fine, but he didn't want to see any color in it. She gave him the thumbs up and ran off to play.

Things were going pretty good, School was in full swing, and she was in Tara Osterhout's 4th grade class. She done a little better in 4th grade than she did in 3rd grade as far as being able to stay in school. She did miss some, actually I thought it was a lot but they told me that she was fine and assured me she was keeping up with the other classmates. For the entire year she got one B and the rest were A's. So she did do well.

The principal told me not to worry, with the grades she was making, with the condition she was in, still taking chemo, her missing one or two days a week would not be a big deal.

Lacey decided she wanted to have a toy drive, to give toys away at St. Francis Hospital. She put an ad in the newspaper, from the first week of October till the week before Christmas. She wanted EVERYONE to know where they could drop the donated toys off. We went to American Appliance in Cushing to get a couple of refrigerator boxes. They only had one so we went looking for another. We found one at the Rent to Own store, there in Cushing. They gave us a recliner box.

We brought them home and wrapped them in Christmas paper. We took one box to Bradley Elementary and the other to the grocery store.

Once again we witnessed an abundant amount of generosity. We even had people give money, so the girls, Lacey and Sarah, could experience going shopping for the toy drive themselves. They had a blast! They bought remote control cars, baby dolls, and all sorts of good stuff. We also bought a bunch of batteries too, to put in the remote control cars and the other toys that needed batteries. They really did have a great time.

My grandmother made Lacey a Santa bag.
I had gone and bought some red flannel material and a white rope to tie the bag with, so she would have something to carry all the toys in, from room to room. Grandma actually made two bags. I had

enough material for two, one bag was Lacey's size and the other, well, lets just say Greg HAD to carry it. I think all four of us could have stepped into it and pulled it over our heads and tied ourselves in it.

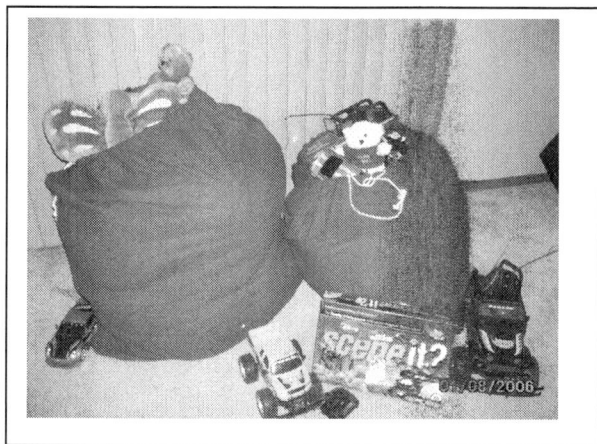

Chapter 10.
Christmas and Excitement

On Christmas morning, we got up pretty early, and we had our family Christmas. The girls opened up their own presents under the tree. Then, we got around, loaded up both bags. Not all of the toys would fit in the two bags. Greg had a ¾ ton, short wide, quad cab, dodge pickup, we filled every crack and cranny of that truck, inside and out. When we got to the hospital, Lacey and I went to the information desk to see if we could get a couple of carts to haul all these toys around. They gave us a cart and an oversized wheelchair. We weren't able to fit all the toys on our little caravan but we put the rest of the toys in the cab of the truck and decided we'd make another trip if we needed to.

We went to the second floor, the same floor where Lacey had stayed, so many times before. We had enough toys to give two toys to each child and their siblings who were there with them. I think we even gave a coloring book to several of the parents too.

I remember when we were in the hospital for Christmas of '05, it was overwhelming, the generosity that we felt from total strangers. But to be on the giving end was the most amazing thing we had ever experienced so far. The feeling you get from doing something for someone else is so much better than when you are on the receiving end.

The first part of December there was a lady from OSU that called, and wanted to see if Lacey would be interested in being a part of the half time show during "Coaches vs. Cancer Swish Night" in both, the women, and the men's game.

If I am not mistaken, I believe the women's game was in January. We were to sell tickets, like we did for the Drillers game, and like the Drillers game, I can't even began to tell you who all went. I know there was a bunch.

They had called and invited Lacey to basketball practice, so that she could meet the players and run through what was going to take place, the night of the game. That was fun, to get to see those girls practice. Some of them were so tall. Greg's youngest son Matthew, and his girlfriend Sara, came with us. They seemed to really enjoy it also.

The night of the game they put us right on the front row. We had never been to a college basketball game before and we loved it. Sometimes, the squeals of they're tennis shoes on the floor, was so loud, it almost hurt your ears, and the way they could jump, oh my goodness, I was just blown away!

A couple of days before the men's game, the coaches wanted us to meet them at Eskimo Joe's. There was a bunch of people going there to eat, in celebration of the big game, and they wanted to walk around with Lacey at the restaurant, to introduce her to some of the more affluent people who were going to be dining there that night. I have a feeling that the coaches wanted these people to see Lacey, and the other children that had been invited that night, up close, to meet them face to face, and have the children tell them a little bit about themselves and their cancer. This way, when the time came to donate during the half time show, these folks would reach a little deeper into their pockets.

Even though we had just been there a few weeks ago for the women's game, when we got there we were lost, we had no idea where they wanted us to go. There were so many people; I had never seen so many people packed into one building. I got a little taste of what Greg feels in crowds, because I was getting nervous.

The people made a lot bigger deal out of the men's game than they did the women's game, which I personally don't think is right. The women ought to be just as important as the men, and they should make a big deal out of both the men and the women's games.

When we first got there we stood in some lobby, which had this memorial thing set up for the ones that had gotten killed on the airplane a year or two earlier. It was really neat, it talked about the players and their lives and their accomplishments at OSU. There were also pictures of former OSU students that had gone on and become famous for whatever reasons, and some history about the university.

We also were able to see Dr. K, there in the lobby, and someone else from the hospital was there, but I can't remember whom. It might have been Jana.

Finally a lady came and told us they were ready for all the kids and their families and friends up stairs. (They told both of the girls they could bring some friends with them, Lacey took Kylie Cusner and Sarah took Avi Overstreet).

Up the stairs, there were glassed in areas, which of course, were for affluent people, or important people, purchased every year. In these areas, they're where couches and comfy chairs, a TV, a refrigerator and a bar, stocked with liquor, of course. In the front of the glassed in areas, there was a sliding glass door that you could walk out onto a balcony and set in the auditorium. They had food catered in, and the owners of the first class areas, invited us to make ourselves at home. They also had all you could eat hotdogs, hamburgers, and ice cream. It was amazing, and we really did enjoy ourselves.

When it came time for the half time show, Greg walked down to the floor with Lacey and they introduced each of the kids, what type of cancer they had, who their parents were, where they lived, where they took treatments, and whether or not they were in remission and how long.

Lacey, got to sit on Big Country's shoulders and shoot baskets. It was really fun for her. After the half time show, Big Country came up to the area we were in, with Lacey, and she introduced him, to all her family and friends. When Big Country stuck out his hand to shake Greg's hand, Big Country's hand swallowed Greg's hand, and Greg has huge hands himself. It was really, really fun for us, and we appreciated it very much.

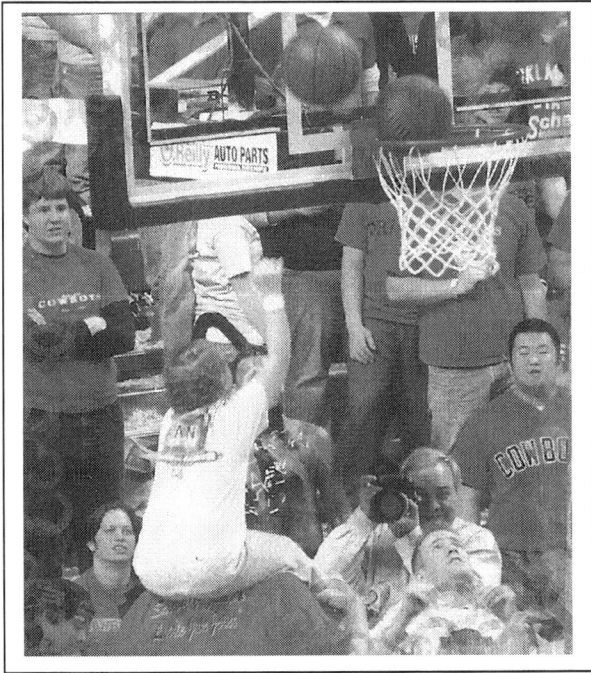

Chapter 11.
Baseball, and Make a Wish

It's softball season again and Lacey's doing so much better this year than she did the last. She's physically stronger, but still not able to run very good because of all the spinal taps she'd had, but she sure put out a good effort. Wyatt didn't put her at the catchers position very much during this year, because I think he was afraid that she'd get hurt, as she was playing fast pitch for the first time that year, and with her having the port, I think Wyatt was being protective of her, but of course she didn't see it that way. She wanted to play catcher and he always put her in the outfield where there's very little action, and she hated that!

The Make-a-wish trip was approaching, and Lacey had seen a set of luggage that she had fallin' in love with. They were at a little boutique shop in Drumright. I went in to see how much they wanted for the luggage, as I thought I might get them as a surprise, if I could afford them. I don't even remember now, how much she was asking for them, but I do remember they were out of the price range I was willing to pay. I also didn't know it, but one of the ladies that worked in the office, at the Vo-Tech, Kathy, overheard the conversation I had with the boutique lady.

Everyone in town knew that we were getting ready for Lacey's Make-A-Wish trip. Kathy followed me outside, and stopped me. She begged me not to buy the luggage, because she had a bunch of luggage that they very rarely used, and she said we could barrow some of hers. I told her I really appreciated the offer, but I'd be afraid of something happening to her luggage, even if it were not our fault, of course we would feel responsible for it and wouldn't have the money to replace it. I thanked her for the offer, and sadly and politely declined.

A few weeks later, Kathy, from the Vo-Tech, called and asked me to come to the Vo-Tech as soon as I had the time, preferably that day, as she said she had something for our family. I asked her what it was and she said, "Well, you'll just have to come see for yourself." The girls and I, loaded up and headed up there. Kathy had told a bunch of teachers and office ladies and gentlemen that we were in need of luggage for our trip. They pooled money together and bought us a 5-peace luggage set, a nice one too, they all have wheels and handles.

I had been promising the girls for months that I would quite smoking when we went on our trip. Greg wasn't comfortable with leaving his truck at the airport parking lot for a week so we asked my mother if she'd take us to the airport, and then leave his truck at their house. Mom didn't allow smoking in her car, so I took my last drag off of my cigarette, right before I got into her car to go to the airport, June 5, 2007.

Chapter 12.
Finally on our way

We were all very nervous, as we had never flown before. Well, I had, but I was to young to remember it. We had never been through security before and we were not aware that we'd have to take off our shoes and socks, unload everything we had in our pockets, and in our carry on bags. We didn't have anything to hide, so it wasn't really that big of a deal, except for the fact that it was time consuming. Finally we got through security and we were looking for our gate number. Because we had never been to an airport before, we didn't have a clue about what we were doing. I asked someone else, what to do, and I'm sure they thought we were quite the hillbillies. We finally found our gate, and waited for our flight to load. It took a while, and we stood and watched a few planes land and take off, and it was pretty neat. Everyone around us could tell that we were first timers, because we kept ooohing and ahhhing at everything.

They finally called out our fight number, and we began to aboard our plane. We were so excited and yet so scared at the same time. It took a little while for all the passengers to get settled, then it moved. We slowly moved away from the loading ramp, and started down the runway. Greg and one of the girls, sat behind me and the other one. As soon as the wheels lifted off the ground, I grabbed Greg's pant leg, down around his ankle, and let out a squeal. Before I could contain myself, I had tears running down my face, but once we were in the air, all was ok.

We flew from Tulsa, to Memphis, in less than an hour. We were supposed to have an hour and a half layover in Memphis, so we found the gate where we were to load for our next fight, and I stayed there, while Greg and the girls went to find us something to eat. When they got back, we were handing out the meals, set down to eat and they called our fight number, to board the plane. We just looked at each other, wrapped our sandwiches up and loaded the plane.

I told the fight attendant that we hadn't had a chance to eat since breakfast, and that we had bought hamburgers and fries in the terminal, and would we be allowed to eat them on the plane? She told us that all we needed to do was wait until we were in the air.

It took less than two hours to get to Florida from Tennessee, but I don't remember what time it was when we got there. When we got off the plane, the resort we stayed at had a man standing with a sign that read "Lacey Rodgers" written on it. He was Swedish I think, and his name was Ed. Very nice guy. He helped us get to our rented vehicle that the Make-a-Wish foundation had arranged for us, and lead us out of the airport parking lot. When we got to the turn off, where we were suppose to go, he points us in the direction to go. He also gave us a map so we could find our way to our resort. Give Kids the World was like stepping into a fairy tale book, as the characters of the book came to life, right before our very eyes.

Most of the people who worked at Give Kids the World, were volunteers. When we first got there, we had to check in at the front office, and while we were waiting to check in, we were looking at the neat pictures that were on the walls. They told us that they were going to have a group meeting for all the new guests at a curtain time, and that only one parent had to come.

When they gave us our key to our Villa, they also gave us a map of the Village, so we would be able to find our way around. Our Villa was circled on the map, and we were able to drive right to it. We weren't allowed to drive our vehicles around the Village, but they provided a train that you could call, to come pick you up and take you anywhere in the Village you wanted to go. The resort was laid out like a little Village, and each of the streets lead to different areas of the Village. These streets were named after former guests that had passed away. When we got to our Villa, everyone grabbed a couple of bags and went inside. Oh my goodness! It had more square footage than our house back home. It was equipped with a fully functional kitchen; a living room that was nice and a big couch, love seat, a couple of chairs and a bigger TV than we had at home. The main bathroom was small, one sink, toilet, and a tub with showerhead. The girls' bathroom was HUGE! Two sinks, one toilet, a whirlpool tub, monster huge, and a shower that had four showerheads!

Greg's bedroom, and mine had a king sized bed. It was so nice. I wanted to take it back home with us.

After we got the Villa all checked out, Greg had about 2 hours before the meeting started, so we decided to walk around the resort for a while and check things over. When we checked in, they gave Lacey a little gold star with her name on it, and the date. They told her to take the gold star to the Magic Castle and the volunteers there would tell her what to do, with her golden star. She was so excited she couldn't wait to take her gold star to the Magic Castle. So off we went to the Magic Castle. There they told her to put her star in this little box, so she did. After a couple of seconds, the box began to rattle and shake. We all took a step back, not real sure what to expect. Then a laser light finally flickered and a little fairy appeared on a TV screen on the wall. Lacey's name was on the star, so the fairy called her by name, and then she introduced herself. She interacted with Lacey for a little while and then told her that if she would come back to the Magic Castle at a certain time the next day, that her star would magically appear on the ceiling of the Magic Castle.

We looked up at the ceiling at this time and there were thousands, hundreds of thousands of little gold stars on the ceiling. The fairy told Lacey that a card, with directions on how to locate her star, would appear on the kitchen table in our Villa.

Inside the Magic Castle, there were other neat things to do also. They had a magical pillow-making factory; where both of the girls got a pillow. Then there was the magical cave, the magical playroom, but neither one of the girls were real interested in that, as it was a little too childish for them. The magical grandfather clock, the magical mirror, there was this ring, that they stuck their faces in, and they appeared in the mirror as the king or queen. Then there was the magical wishing well, and so many other very cool things, that are just too numerous to mention.

It was time for the meeting so I took the girls back to the Villa, let them change into their swimsuits, and walked them back down to the pool. They played until Greg got out of his meeting, and it was starting to get dark so we all went back to the Villa.

We set the alarm for 7am. After we were ready, we walked to the gingerbread house to eat breakfast.

At the gingerbread house, there are many displays of things sent from former kids parents that are donated to, "Give Kids the World", articles of all kinds of things that were from children that had died from various illnesses.

Anyway, after we got through eating, we called Robert and Christle and the boys, and they were waiting for us at the front gate of Magic Kingdom. We parked our van, then followed the crowd. Magic Kingdom is situated on an island. In order to get to the island we had a choice, we could take a trolley, (it's kind of like a train only it runs on one rail not two), or we could take the fairy across, and we chose the fairy.

As we approached Magic Kingdom, it looked just like it does on TV, but the closer we got the more amazing it became. Christle and the boys spotted us before we spotted them. The boys were so excited to show the girls around. Of course, this was the second or third time they'd been to Disney World. Finally we were off to venture Magic Kingdom. It was so awesome! The first thing we saw, was a barbershop quartet, oh they were so good. We danced in the street with them. I could have stood there for a lot longer than we did.

At our resort, they gave Lacey a necklace with a badge clipped to it that let EVERYONE know that she was a Make-a-Wish child. Everyone treated us like we were royalty. We never had to stand in line, when the person at the front gate saw Lacey's badge they would ask how many were in our group and they took us directly to the front of the line.

I remember this one guy, I'm sure he had been drinking some and just being a smarty pants, but he says to us, "why do you guys get to cut in front of everyone else?" I told him he had to have a child with a life threatening disease like cancer or something like that. Of course when I told him that he apologized and you could tell he felt bad for mouthing off. The whole day was so great! There were so many things that we did I can't even remember them all. I just remember we had a blast and we did not want the day to come to an end.

We were all getting very tired, and Robert and Christle wanted to show us they're resort. We all took the trolley, but then when we got to the van Greg and I got off the trolley and took the van to their resort. The girls wanted to go with them.

Their resort was pretty cool. They stayed at the Pops Central (I think that was the name) the thyme to the whole place was 50's music. It was really neat. We were all hungry so we went down to the resorts restaurant. It was like stepping in a time machine and going back to the 50's. The waitresses wore roller skates to serve you at your table.

After we ate Robert and Christle showed us around a little bit, took us up to their room. It was getting late and we were all tired, and they were leaving the next day. So we said our good byes, and went back to our room. We got baths, watched a little TV and went to bed.

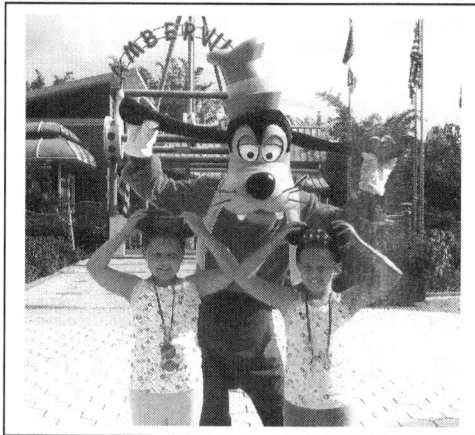

Chapter 13.
To the beach, and then home

One of the things we sure did not want to miss was going to the beach. Getting there, was very exiting, and I am sure the girls would love to tell you about it sometime, but for now, we will skip the details.

We found a clean spot on the beach to spread out all our towels. I set on the towels for a little bit while Greg and the girls went on out to the water. I took some video and pictures of them playing in the ocean but then after a little while, I just couldn't take it any longer; I had to get out there with them and have some fun. The waves weren't to bad, but there were a couple of times we would be standing on the bottom of the ocean floor, look up, and see this wave coming over the top of our heads and swish us up toward the beach. It was great!

One wave grabbed Lacey's goggles and ripped them off her face. She was ok, but just a little sad, as she had lost her brand new goggles.

After about 3 hours we were tired and sunburned, so we decided to head back to Kissimmee, that's the little town our resort was in.

When we got back to the resort we looked on the scheduled events the resort was having that night and the girls were excited to learn they were having a fishing tournament.

We got all the sand wash off, and found something to eat, and we were off to the pond.

Then they played some games. They split up into groups, and one member of the group was a candy cane. The other members wrapped them in red and white crape paper. They had to see which team could do it the fastest.

After that they sang and danced in the streets. Even the president of Give Kids the World danced with Lacey and Sarah. Our last night was very memorable. We'll never forget it!

When we returned to the Villa, we got all our things together and ready to go to the airport. Our vacation was over, and we had a blast! When we checked out they gave us a packet that included: a CD of pictures, that the resort photographer had taken, a passport that had different amusement parks and museums in it that had to be used 1 year within the date of our departure, which was June 11, 2007.

We followed the map backwards, which they had given us at the airport, when we had first arrived. We were tired and a little sad that we had to go home so soon, but thankful that we had the opportunity to experience all these things. On the airplane back home I was thinking about all the things we had experienced and seen, but most of all, I was thanking God for all the blessings He had granted us. As I was thinking about all of this, I was reminded of a story I had heard, a long time ago, about a man who asked God if he could have a different cross to bare. The Lord told him, "Come with me, my child and bring your cross." The Lord took this man to a room full of crosses. All of these crosses were different shapes and sizes, big ones, little ones, short fat ones, tall skinny ones, and in every color imaginable. There were shelves full of crosses, Crosses hanging on the walls and even off the ceiling. Crosses were everywhere this man turned. Finally, after careful consideration, the man decided upon the cross he wanted. "Ok Lord this is it, this is the cross I want." The Lord turned to the man, gently laid his hand on his shoulder, smiled and said, " My child, that is the cross you were carrying when you came to me."

I feel like God has given Greg and I the opportunity to walk that room of crosses. Give Kids the World, was kind of like, that room full of crosses. Everywhere we turned, everywhere we walked we could see a bigger, heavier cross to bear. Give Kids the World, was created for children who had life threatening diseases, and they're families. There were children at Give Kids the World, that couldn't walk and run. Some, you could snap your fingers in front of they're faces and they wouldn't even know you were there.

I quickly realized, no matter how heavy our cross might be, it could be a lot heavier. I began to cry and thank God for our cross. No matter how heavy our cross is, we will bear that cross until God sees fit to relieve us, of that cross.

When our plane landed in Tulsa, my sister Christle and her two boys were waiting to take us back to Mom and Dads where our truck was.

When we got there, we unloaded the luggage from Christle's van to Greg's truck. We did take in our souvenir bag to show everyone the things we brought back with us. We set and visited for a while, told everyone about our trip, and how much fun we'd had, and some of the things we had seen. We also had a souvenir for Mom and Dad from the girls. We were tired and decided to go home to rest up, because Greg had to go back to work the next day. We unloaded all of our things out of the truck into the house, and then unloaded the suitcases. We put the dirty clothes in the laundry to start washing. After starting a load of laundry, we finished unpacking everything else.

The Make-a-Wish foundation sent a disposable camera with us to take pictures for their new brochures. I put the camera in the envelope provided with the camera, (stamped and self addressed), and got it ready to mail the next day.

We felt very blessed that Greg was able to work when we got back because it rained off and on most of the summer. I don't think it quit raining till after the 4th of July. It was so wet and sloppy that we were unable to have our annual 4th celebration out at my Mom and Dad's that year, plus, my grandmother was out in her back yard playing ball with my little cousin and twisted her ankle on the wet grass and broke it.

Lacey continued a light dose of chemo everyday by mouth, and would for another 9 months. It didn't make her sick very often, but we did notice that if she didn't get plenty of sleep at night, that she would become ill. I always made sure she went to bed a little early, whether it was a school night or not. Some of the time; I had to fuss with her a little, because she did not like the idea of not being able to stay up on weekends. She can be quit the night owl if I'd let her.

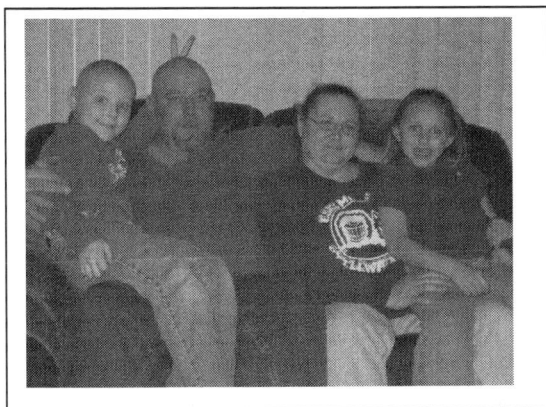

Chapter 14.
Starting 5th Grade

Her 5th grade year went pretty smoothly. Nothing out of the ordinary happened, and she was becoming a normal little girl again. Her teacher was Mrs. Kates and she loved her class very much. Lacey's class got a new student, and her name was Stormy Kellogg. Lacey and Stormy hit it off real well. Stormy invited Lacey over to her house to spend the night, and Lacey met Stormy's little foster sister, Monique. Lacey and Monique had something in common they both had cancer. Monique's cancer was different than Lacey's, a lot more aggressive. Lacey and Monique and the entire family developed closeness right away. Lacey loved Monique and the Kellogg family very much.

I'm not exactly sure what month it was, but someone had contacted us to see if we'd be interested in doing an interview for the radio. They were doing a tribute to the Make-a-wish foundation, trying to encourage people to donate to the foundation. They were trying to get people to interview with them, about their Make-a-wish experience. We had just come home from our trip a few months before, so it was all real fresh. We had never been inside a radio station before, so they gave a tour and showed us where and how they do it all, and we found it very fascinating.

The way they edited the interview was amazing, and they made it sound so neat! They even put it on a CD for us, so we would be able to listen to it anytime we wanted. I didn't actually hear it on the radio the day they aired it, but Lacey's 3rd grade teacher heard it. (her teacher, when she was first diagnosed). She was crying when she called, and said it was amazing and that she really needed that today. You see, not to long before this all happened, they had found out that her nephew, Cody Paul's cancer, had relapsed and he was going another round with chemo. This radio interview with Lacey hit her pretty hard.

It's Lacey's favorite time of the year again, softball season. Bret Fluellen was the coach that year, and for some reason that team didn't have the catcher's gear. I told Bret, that if Lacey were to be the primary catcher, I would go to Academy and buy the gear for her. She had played that position, ever since T-ball, and she was good at it and that was the position she preferred.

Bret knew she was good at that position and agreed to put Lacey at catcher. She was so excited! We went to Academy and got all the gear she needed; the helmet, the chest protector, the shin guards, the knee savers, and the catcher's glove. ($265) Then we bought her new cleats. (That is the shoe that you wear, when you are playing baseball, so you don't slip).

Lacey had been talking about how good her softball team was this year, to everyone in the clinic. Dr. K decided he wanted to watch her play. Lacey told him that the Mannford game would be the closest they'd get to Tulsa, so she told him the day and time of the game, and he did show up. Lacey was so excited. He said he'd never been to one of his patients' games before, and that he really enjoyed it. He was unable to stay for the whole game but it was nice that he got to come for a little bit, anyway. I know it made Lacey very happy.

In March of 2008 we finally found a house to buy. We had been praying for God to deliver us from the worn out old house we were living in. Our little realtor lady, Kelly, had been so patient with us. Time after time she'd show us a house, and it seemed like for whatever reason, something just wouldn't seem right. Kelly looked and looked for us a house, for about 5 or 6 years.

One day she calls me and wants us to look at this house that had come on the market, just one hour before she called me. She knew Greg and told him he did not have a week to think about this one, because it wouldn't last the week.

We went to look at the house, Lacey wasn't feeling good that day and was out of school, and so she went with us to look. We all fell in love with the house. They were asking $36,500, for the house, it was in foreclosure. We offered them $35,500., and later that evening, I called Kelly to see if we could take Sarah, and my Mom and Dad over to see it. Kelly had told me she was just fixing to call me; she'd just gotten off the phone with the bank that had the house, and it would be ok if we went to see OUR new house.

I asked her, "What do you mean OUR new house?" She said, "They've accepted your offer, the house is yours." I went to my knees and started to cry hysterically. Greg thought there was something wrong. When I told him they accepted our offer, he got this look on his face, like someone had just kicked him really hard. The girls started screaming and jumping up and down! I told Kelly, "Don't play with me Kelly. Are you serious?" Kelly said, "Delinda I would not do that, as I know how long you and your family have been waiting for this. The house is yours."

When I got off the phone I called Mom and Dad, and Grandma and Grandpa and Aunt Wanda. Everyone met us at our new house. They were all so excited and happy for us. God is so good; He blessed us with a beautiful home. (3 bedrooms, & 2 baths) I love it and I'm so happy!

On April 11, 2008 Lacey took her last chemo pills. She was finished! Well, with chemo anyway. They still wanted us to go to the clinic once a month for blood counts for the first year after stopping chemo. They say if the cancer relapses, most generally it will do so in the first year after stopping the chemo.

Chapter 15.
No More Chemo

Lacey wanted to have a NO MORE CHEMO party. We actually had two, one at the church for our Church Family, to share in her victory, where we had cake, which Sis. Sherri Smith done a wonderful job on it, and then we had ice cream and soda's. The Porter boys brought their guitars, and we set around and sang Gospel songs. Then we had a party at the park in Drumright for our community to share in her victory. A few of the young folks from the church, came over for it, Bro. Brad Bell, The two Martin Girls, India and Alexis and another boy but I didn't know. We advertised the party for several weeks. And had a pretty good turn out.

Tara Osterhout and Shelly Martin borrowed the slushy machine from the school and made slushies for us, and Keidra made a huge cake. One of the guys that works with Greg, brought his PA system over and we played music and also played the radio interview for

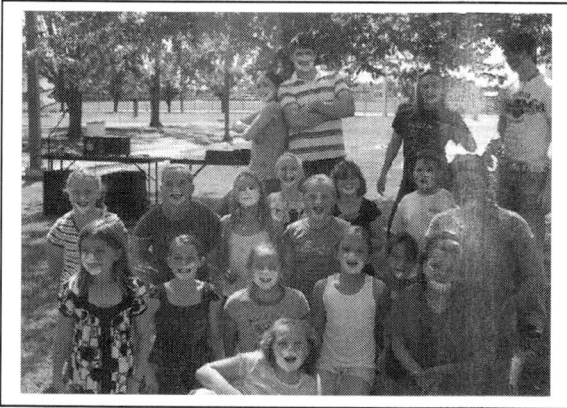

everyone to hear. We played games, and some brought gifts, for Lacey. It really was a lot of fun.

Sometime during the month of October, 2008, I seen Dr. Erin Trippy, in a consignment store here in Drumright. I walked up to her and asked if she remembered me, because we hadn't seen her since that very first time we had taken Lacey to the Drumright Emergency Room.

She looked at me kind of funny and said, " Well, I know I probably should know you, but I'm not sure." I told her who I was and she gave me a great big hug and began to cry. She asked me, " Do you have any idea what a miracle Lacey is?"
I told her, " Yes ma'am I think we do."

She told me that she had always believed in miracles, but had never personally experienced one until that night. She said she had called everyday to check on Lacey, and was astonished every time one of the nurses at St. Francis pediatric Oncology, would tell her that Lacey was doing so much better.

Dr. Trippy told me that she truly did not believe we would be bringing her home. She thought she was too far-gone, even for St. Francis to save her. There again God proved, that He was the one in charge.

They talked about removing her port during spring break. But she quickly vetoed that idea. That was right at the beginning of her softball season and she didn't want to take the chance of something going wrong and not being able to play.

They decided on the end of the season somewhere around the end of July. This way, she would have 2 or 3 weeks before school started, to heal, and then start training for school softball.

They scheduled Lacey to have an echo done at the end of June. An echo is a scan of her heart to make sure there were no blood clots in any of the veins or vessels going to or coming from her heart, so that when they do remove her port, the blood clot (if any) wouldn't go to her head and kill her.

The echo turned out normal, so then we scheduled a consultation meeting with the surgeon on July 23, 2009. The surgeon doing the operation was Dr. Mary Li (Lee). We had a pre-op scheduled the same afternoon, at St. Francis. Don't ask me what a pre-op is because I don't understand it and they even explained it to me and I still don't understand.

My Mom went with me to these appointments, as Greg needed to work, and the office that we had to go to was down town Tulsa. I don't know my way around, so I didn't want to go by myself.

Dr. Li told Lacey she could not swim, emerge herself in bath water, or even sweat for 2 weeks after the surgery.

After the appointment we had about two hours until it was time for us to go to St. Francis for her next appointment. Greg's cousin Terry, opened a new Shiloes restaurant, and the grand opening was that day, so we went to eat there. Christle, my sister, and her youngest son, Matthew met us there and we had lunch together. We were expecting our next appointment to take an hour and a half, that's what they told us to expect, but it only took about 45 minutes. I'm glad it didn't take as long as they said it would.

This was on a Thursday so Lacey had to put up with the port for another 3 days. They scheduled her operation for Monday, July 27, 2009 at 8:15 am. They told us to be there by 7am. I wanted to take the girls to the water park in Cushing, as Lacey only had 3 days to swim and have fun till her port was to be removed, then it would be pretty much couch time for a week and total boredom the next. Things didn't workout for us to go to the water park on Friday, but Greg had to work on Saturday so I promised them we would go on Saturday. Then on Sunday, we went to church, and they announced that Lacey was having her port removed the next day (Monday) and requested prayer. On our way home from church, Jeremy, Keidra, Jarrett, and Kristi wanted to know if they could go swimming out at my Mom and Dads. Lacey wanted to go swimming anyway, because after tomorrow, she wouldn't get to go swimming for 2 weeks, and today, she's got someone to swim with. After everyone got tired of swimming, we got out, got dressed and went home. We had to go to bed early because we had to get up at 5 am. Sarah went to her big sisters house to spend the night because she didn't want to spend a lot of time waiting in the waiting room at the hospital. 5 o'clock came way to soon. We left the house by 6 am and got to the hospital by 7 am. I do not understand why they wanted us to be there by 7 am, as we sat in the waiting room till 9 am anyway. Then, when they finally called her back to prep her for operation they gave her something to calm her nerves and she got pretty goofy by the time they made us leave the room. 79.

About 1 hour later, they came and got us out of the waiting room, and the surgeon went over with us again what to do if this or that happened. She said Lacey done real good, and that she was pretty looped when they brought her back. The nurse began to tell Lacey what they were going to do and Lacey interrupted the nurse and said, "I know, your going to take the port out, then Dr. K is going to give me a spinal tap and a bone marrow." The nurse said, "Yes, your right, you saved me some breath." They took us back to the recovery room and when we first seen her, her eyes were opened. Right away she recognized us both, she kind of gave us a half smile and then moaned. Then she went right back to sleep for a few minutes.

One of the nurses handed Greg her port. We tried to wake Lacey to show her the port. She halfway woke, and said, "Daddy, I wanna see." He tried to show it to her but she just couldn't keep her little eyes open long enough to look at it. Greg was standing next to her bed talking to the nurse and trying to talk to Lacey, to wake her up a little and I was texting all our friends and family, to let them know she was out of surgery and doing great!

They moved her from the recovery room to a private room and it didn't take very long for her to be on her feet and ready to get out of there. She hadn't eaten since super the night before, and it was almost 1o'clock. She wanted to go back to Shiloes to eat, so we did.

Lacey slept most of the way home. By the time we got home it was 3:30 pm and the pain medication they gave her in the hospital was wearing off, and she was hurting pretty bad! I gave her the pain pills they prescribed for her, and she stayed home with Greg, while I went to get Sarah at Jim and Shelly Martins.

Sarah's softball team was having they're end of the season softball party. When I got there, Shelly told me Lacey's wonderful friend Monique, had passed away that morning, (July 27, 2009).

I started to cry when Shelly had told me about Monique, and I knew that Lacey would be heart broken. Lacey was aware that Monique was in really bad condition, and that the doctors hadn't given her long, but they were such good buddies.

That night, Lacey asked us to pray for her, as she was afraid she might roll over on her left side and hurt the incision. So, we all prayed for her. The next morning, the first thing out of her mouth was, "Thank you Jesus!" Because she realized she hadn't rolled over on her left side all night.

She had been up for a couple of hours before she decided she needed a pain pill. Which I thought was a blessing, because God was having mercy on her and she didn't seem to need the pain pills.

My Mom and I went to Bro. Bill and Sis. Marcelle's, and I cleaned and Mom took care of Sis. Marcelle. The girls stayed with their Papa. Lacey didn't need a pain pill till after we got back home at 5:00 pm.

She had been extremely bored and not happy about having to stay on the couch, as she's always been so active, and not used to doing nothing at all.

On the next day, Wednesday July 29 2009, I had to go to Sapulpa to set with Bro. Glenn, so that Sis. Sadie could go take care of business in town. Lacey went with me. She didn't ask for a pain pill till 2 pm so I knew she was doing much better.

On the day of her follow up appointment I had a really bad day.

1. I found out I was $150 over drawn.
2. I got a flat tire on the way.
3. I got lost on the way to the appointment.
4. When we left the appointment I got lost again.
5. When we went to eat lunch, I locked the keys in my car.

Something else happened after we got home but for the life of me I cannot remember what it was, but her appointment went real good, and Dr. Li said she could not ask for it to look any better.

It's over! Finally God has seen us through our worst nightmare, our Perfect Cross and we survived. Only by the grace of God, we survived. I truly do understand that saying now, "What you think is going to kill you, just seems in the end, to just make you stronger."

The End
Author: Delinda Rodgers

Extra things:

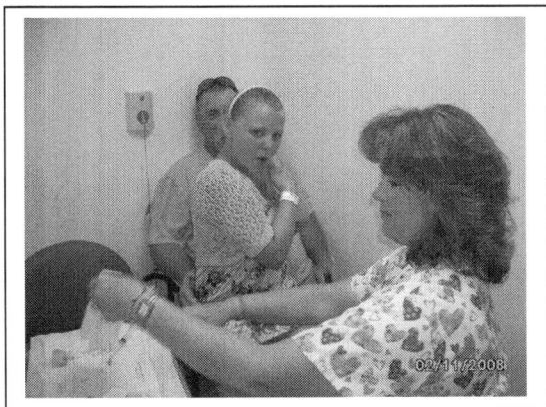

Picture of the final Checkup

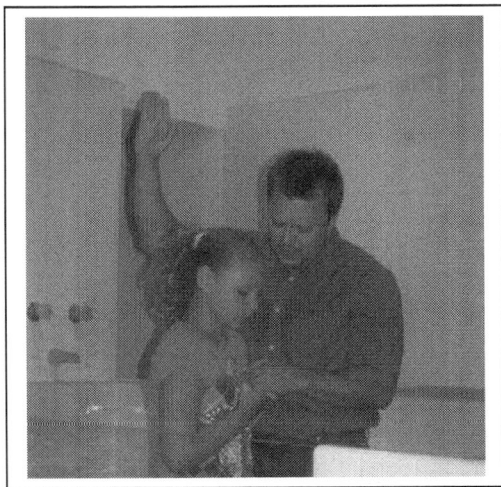

Lacey was baptized on July 11, 2010